# A Carolina Path to Regenerative Farming:

## 2025 White Papers, Essays and Practical Models

## Editor's Introduction

This booklet is my tangible hope in your hands, a hope to start fruitful conversations and get to work regenerating our land, culture, and society. For growing a better future, I and my family and friends are not proposing an abstract model; rather, in these pages we're inviting you to walk with us as we continue to test out a living one.

In America generally, and in the rural Southeast especially, there is much that needs to be regenerated. Political polarization is only one dramatic symptom of things amiss. In order to attain a bright outlook in this region, many areas must be restored or revived. A thoughtful observer will sense that any good way forward may involve healthy farm livelihoods, vibrant rural communities, and resilient local food systems. We might best begin the good work by fertilizing the human mind, and that work of fertilizing is the chief purpose of this booklet.

You will find these pages led and anchored by a triad of white papers, one presented in a modified APA style and two in modified CSE format (based on their topics and tones). Supplemented less formally by a few related articles, the collection then concludes with a policy brief which comes full circle to give abbreviated action steps suggested from the white papers. Here is an even more brief nutshell summary.

- **Problem**: *declining farm viability, degraded soils and ecosystems, and growing social distress*
- **Opportunity**: *rebuilding foundations of resilience by shifting cropland acreage to agroforestry*
- **Why chestnuts**: *durable, storable, calorie-rich food staple with many layers of long-term benefits*
- **Policy & market plan**: *empower farmers to begin making this shift to regional sustainability*

The multilayered nature of intertwined challenges faced by our children's generation demands generating solutions through a well-researched and thorough but urgent process. So, here we present you with some fruits of such a process, hopefully given in a professional, detailed and substantial enough way to merit practical consideration. A transparent look at our process and these papers' authorship – The DeepRichDirt Project – can be found at www.wagramorchard.com/deeprichdirt. Also on that page, *this material is available for free download.* **This is not copyrighted or claimed as intellectual property. We welcome free use, copying, and sharing of this product.**

Taken together, my team and I hope that this booklet in its entirety includes all the key initial pieces to begin a productive series of conversations and interrelated efforts or partnerships, establishing a compelling case of how we can bring durable improvement to our homeland.

*Nate Crew*

# CONTENTS

# PAPER 1:

# BRANCHES OF HEALING

## Chestnut Cultivation and the Renewal of Mind, Meaning, and Belonging

## Executive Summary — Key Insights and Recommendations

*Overview*

This paper explores how chestnut cultivation can serve as a practical and symbolic pathway toward mental, ecological, and cultural renewal in the United States — especially across the Carolinas, where rural decline, soil depletion, and social fragmentation intersect. It argues that reintroducing chestnut groves into working and community landscapes can help mend the modern disconnection between humans and their living environments, restoring both ecological balance and psychological coherence.

At its heart, the paper invites a paradigm shift: from extraction to participation, from isolation to belonging. By planting and tending chestnuts, individuals and communities can recover a sense of purpose grounded in the slow, enduring rhythms of the natural world.

*Key Insights*

• Healing Through Reciprocity: Working with perennial tree crops like chestnuts cultivates patience, presence, and responsibility — countering the attention fragmentation and alienation characteristic of modern life.

• Ecological Regeneration as Therapy: The same actions that restore ecosystems (planting, tending, observing growth) foster neural and emotional repair, offering low-cost and high-impact interventions for trauma, depression, and disconnection.

• Cultural Renewal: The chestnut's story — loss, adaptation, and return — mirrors the human search for renewal. Its reintroduction and spread can inspire art, storytelling, and creative movements rooted in reciprocity rather than consumption.

• Regional Opportunity: In the Carolinas, where degraded soils and rural disinvestment have left both land and people in need of recovery, chestnut cultivation offers a unifying model for local food systems, therapy initiatives, and regenerative economies.

• Belonging as Infrastructure: True sustainability depends not only on policy or technology but on shared meaning — on communities that see care for the land as care for themselves.

*Recommendations*

• Establish Land-Based Therapeutic Centers — Pilot programs in the Carolinas integrating trauma therapy, veteran reintegration, and regenerative agriculture through chestnut cultivation.

• Fund Creative Agrarian Residencies — Support artists, writers, and filmmakers in residency programs that merge creative practice with ecological stewardship.

• Incorporate Chestnut Ecology into Education — Partner with schools, tribal nations, and local farms to teach ecological literacy, interdependence, and patience through hands-on cultivation.

• Reform Agricultural Incentives — Redirect portions of subsidies from annual commodity crops to perennial systems, helping farmers diversify income and build climate resilience.

• Build Local "Understory Circles" — Encourage community cooperatives and shared groves where neighbors collaborate to plant, harvest, and learn, turning therapy into a practice of tending.

## A Culture in Crisis

Across the United States, the invisible roots of despair have begun to surface. Rising rates of depression, anxiety, addiction, and suicide now mark the contours of a nation struggling to locate meaning within a system that prizes speed, abstraction, and consumption.[1] The causes are manifold — economic precarity, digital isolation, ecological grief — but they share a common substrate: the slow estrangement of human life from the living world.

In earlier generations, to live was to touch the seasons — to know the scent of spring soil, the angle of autumn light, the patience of trees. Today, most Americans encounter food as a packaged commodity, not a product of place; they encounter nature as scenery, not kinship. This disconnection from ecological participation is more than cultural amnesia. Increasing research in psychology, psychiatry, and neuroscience indicates that human wellbeing depends upon reciprocal interaction with natural systems.[2] When that reciprocity is severed, psychic and social disintegration follow.

In the Carolinas, where farmland now alternates with sprawling subdivisions, the crisis manifests in subtle but telling ways: young people who have never grown or foraged anything they eat; veterans transitioning out of military service without a new mission; artists and thinkers seeking grounding in an age of algorithmic churn. The same landscapes that once sustained subsistence agriculture and close-knit communities now often yield only traffic, debt, and disaffection.

*...young people who have never grown or foraged anything they eat; veterans transitioning out of military service without a new mission...*

Yet within this fragmentation lies potential. The work of cultivation — planting, tending, watching, waiting — remains one of humanity's oldest healing arts. When directed toward tree crops such as the chestnut, that work acquires an added dimension: it becomes a long-term act of restoration, feeding both body and psyche while reweaving the bonds between human purpose and ecological process.

Chestnut cultivation stands apart as a living metaphor of resilience. The American chestnut, once dominant in Eastern forests, was nearly eradicated by blight in the early twentieth century. Today, through hybridization and human care, it is returning — slowly, silently, across Appalachian ridges, piedmont fields, and the eastern areas. Its comeback offers not only ecological hope but psychological instruction: that from near-extinction, renewal is possible when roots remain.

This paper explores the chestnut as both therapeutic practice and cultural symbol. It asks what might happen if a society facing disconnection and despair reoriented itself around acts of slow, participatory creation — if healing were pursued not through consumption but through cultivation. In tracing the interdependence of mind and the land, it seeks to demonstrate that the way back to health may begin not in clinics or classrooms, but in the shaded understory where patience and purpose take root, where the soil grows deeper and richer.

## The Psychological Ecology of Modern Life

Modern life unfolds at a pace and scale that the nervous system was never designed to endure.[3] The average person now receives more daily stimuli than an agrarian ancestor would have encountered in an entire year. Attention, once shaped by natural rhythms, is fractured across notifications and feeds. Even moments of rest are colonized by curated noise — visual, auditory, informational.

This overstimulation is paired with profound undernourishment of the senses. The tactile, olfactory, and kinesthetic engagement once central to daily living has largely disappeared. Hands that once dug, pruned, or gathered natural objects now tap glass screens. Bodies calibrated to variation in light, temperature, and texture move through climate-controlled sameness. The result is a population that is mentally crowded but sensorially starved.

Clinical psychology has begun to name this condition in fragments — "nature-deficit disorder," "technostress," "eco-anxiety."[4] Yet these are not isolated pathologies but symptoms of a deeper eco-psychological imbalance: a severing of feedback between inner and outer worlds. When the environment ceases to mirror human continuity — when cycles of birth, death, decay, and renewal are obscured — the psyche loses its primary template for resilience.

*Emerging research supports what indigenous and agrarian cultures long intuited: contact with living systems is essential to human regulation and meaning-making.*

Emerging research supports what indigenous and agrarian cultures long intuited: contact with living systems is essential to human regulation and meaning-making. Time spent in natural settings correlates strongly with reductions in cortisol, improved mood stability, and enhanced executive function.[5] Moreover, acts of stewardship — gardening, forestry, cultivation — compound these benefits by aligning purpose with care, transforming passive exposure into participatory relationship.

Nowhere is this interdependence more evident than in the act of tending trees. A tree is not instant gratification. It demands patience, long horizons, acceptance of growth beyond one's lifespan. To plant a tree is to enter into continuity — a contract between generations. In this way, the psychological ecology of tree cultivation directly counters the accelerative pressures of modernity.

For veterans returning from war, for artists facing creative fatigue, for those recovering from trauma or addiction, the discipline of slow, embodied care offers what few therapies can: a tangible sense of contribution within living time.[6] Cultivation becomes an existential anchor — a way to experience belonging through becoming.

In the Carolinas, where military installations, creative hubs, and rural dislocation coexist within a single region, such practices carry profound relevance. Here, chestnut planting can reconnect fractured communities with enduring landscapes, turning empty fields into living classrooms of patience and possibility. As each sapling extends its roots, it gestures toward a rebalanced psyche — one that no longer seeks control over the world, but communion with it.

## Chestnut as a Living Therapy: Regeneration Through Relationship

Among tree crops, the chestnut occupies a singular position — nutritionally, ecologically, and symbolically. Its nuts, rich in complex carbohydrates yet low in fat, offer a food that nourishes without excess; its canopy provides shade that cools microclimates; its deep roots stabilize and aerate the soil. But beyond its measurable functions, the chestnut extends an invitation: to enter into a long-term partnership of care and co-creation.

In therapeutic contexts, this invitation aligns with growing fields of horticultural therapy, ecotherapy, and trauma-informed land work, all of which recognize that relationship with the living world can catalyze recovery.[7] Chestnut cultivation embodies key principles of these modalities: grounding, rhythm, patience, reciprocity, and future orientation. To nurture a chestnut is to engage in an act of trust — faith that something small will endure and give beyond oneself.

Psychologically, such faith combats what trauma specialists call temporal collapse, the condition in which the past overwhelms the present and future possibility narrows.[8] By contrast, planting a tree reopens the time horizon. It asserts that tomorrow can be different, and that the self can play a part in its cyclical unfolding.

*For veterans and trauma survivors, this shift can be profound.*

For veterans and trauma survivors, this shift can be profound. Clinical studies have shown that structured engagement with land-based projects — especially those involving growth cycles and measurable progress — can reduce PTSD symptoms, improve emotional regulation, and increase social cohesion.[9] When these projects include tree planting, participants report feelings of legacy and belonging that extend beyond individual achievement.[10]

Chestnuts, unlike many crops, require companionship. They do not fruit alone; they rely on cross-pollination. This interdependence models the relational nature of healing itself. Just as no chestnut thrives in isolation, no psyche recovers apart from connection. Working in small groups to tend young orchards can therefore become a practice of mutual restoration: each participant tending both tree and neighbor.

In the eastern and piedmont regions of the Carolinas, where some degraded farmland still remembers the chestnut's ancestral range, such efforts could weave therapy, community, and ecological renewal into a single fabric. Cooperative replanting programs could pair veterans, at-risk youth, or individuals in recovery with environmental educators and farmers, forming living networks of care.

Within these groves, labor and meaning converge. Digging, mulching, watering — these are not mere tasks but rituals of re-entry into life. The earth offers resistance and response; seasons mark progress in visible increments. Over time, the human nervous system begins to entrain to these natural cadences, replacing hypervigilance with attunement, alienation with belonging.

The act of tending thus becomes a mirror for inner regeneration. As the soil thickens, so does patience; as roots deepen, so does presence. The chestnut orchard becomes both habitat and metaphor — a landscape where ecological and psychological recovery proceed in tandem.


## Creative Renewal and Cultural Meaning: The Chestnut as Muse

Every culture is shaped, at least in part, by the plants it reveres. Grain civilizations became empires of uniformity; olive and vine cultures fostered long memory and ritual; forests gave rise to mythologies of transformation. In this lineage, a chestnut culture — if rekindled — might offer something the modern psyche urgently lacks: a grounded poetics of endurance.

The American chestnut's story is one of near-erasure and improbable return. Once towering across the Appalachians, it fed countless species, shaded homesteads, and sustained rural economies. Its sudden disappearance in the early twentieth century — felled by a foreign blight within a human lifetime — left both ecological and psychic scars.[11] For the generations that followed, its absence became an unspoken metaphor for loss: how swiftly abundance can vanish, how fragile continuity can be.

To replant chestnuts is therefore not merely an agricultural act but a creative and mythic gesture. It tells a new story into being — one in which restoration is still possible, and in which humans become active participants in renewal rather than detached observers of decline. For artists, writers, and thinkers, this is fertile symbolic ground. It suggests that beauty and meaning arise not from control but from collaboration with living systems.

Contemporary psychology increasingly acknowledges what poets have always known: that imagination is ecological.[12] When the mind is cut off from the sensory richness of the natural world, creativity withers into repetition; when reconnected, it blossoms into vision. Studies on "biophilic design" and "nature exposure and creativity" confirm that contact with organic forms — trees, flowing water, uneven light — enhances divergent thinking and problem-solving.[13]

In this light, the chestnut orchard becomes a studio, an open-air sanctuary where patience and observation yield inspiration. The slowness of tree growth disciplines the restless imagination, guiding it toward forms that evolve rather than explode. Each season brings subtle revision — buds swelling, leaves returning, hulls hardening — a living tutorial in the art of process.

*The Carolinas, with their layered histories of music, storytelling, and craftsmanship, are poised to reinterpret these lessons.*

The Carolinas, with their layered histories of music, storytelling, and craftsmanship, are poised to reinterpret these lessons. A new creative movement could emerge from ecological re-engagement — painters capturing light through chestnut leaves, filmmakers tracing the arc of a grove across years, songwriters weaving metaphors of root and resilience. Such works might begin to recalibrate collective imagination toward stewardship rather than extraction.

In an era when culture often feels detached from consequence, chestnut cultivation rebinds creation to care. It offers the artist not abstraction but response: the humus underfoot, the arc of a limb, the shared labor of renewal. Through it, beauty is no longer a commodity but a conversation — between mind and matter, maker and soil.

As chestnuts return to the landscape, they carry with them the possibility of cultural coherence — a sense that art, work, and life might once again draw nourishment from the same ground.


## Toward a Culture of Belonging: Recommendations and Vision

If the malaise of modern life stems from severance — from land, from meaning, from one another — then the renewal of health must begin with acts that rebind. Chestnut cultivation offers such an act, uniting personal well-being, ecological repair, and communal purpose within a single gesture of care. But for this vision to take root beyond isolated groves, it must be nurtured by frameworks that recognize the interdependence of psyche, soil, and society.

## 1. Integrative Land-Based Therapy Programs

Governments, universities, and veterans' organizations could collaborate to establish land-based therapeutic centers centered on perennial agriculture. Pilot programs in the Carolinas might combine trauma-informed counseling with chestnut planting, blending horticultural therapy and vocational training.[14] These centers would not only restore landscapes but equip participants with transferable skills in regenerative farming, arboriculture, and ecological design.

## 2. Artistic Residencies and Creative Stewardship

Public and private arts foundations could sponsor creative agrarian residencies — seasonal placements where writers, visual artists, musicians, and filmmakers contribute to and interpret reforestation efforts. By coupling artistic creation with hands-on cultivation, these programs would model a new ethos of creative participation, grounding inspiration in ecological reciprocity.

## 3. Educational Partnerships and Youth Engagement

Incorporating chestnut ecology into school gardens and outdoor curricula can foster early awareness of interdependence and patience. Cooperative programs with local farms and tribal nations might help students witness firsthand how tree crops anchor both ecosystems and economies. A generation raised planting and tasting chestnuts will carry a visceral understanding of time as teacher.

## 4. Incentives for Perennial Transition

Public policy can catalyze transformation by aligning subsidies, grants, and research funding with perennial systems. Redirecting even a fraction of current support for annual monocultures toward tree-based agroforestry would empower farmers to diversify income while sequestering carbon and building resilient soils.[15] In the Carolinas, where many smallholders struggle against volatile commodity markets, such support could anchor both livelihoods and landscapes.

## 5. Networks of Belonging

Finally, community-level initiatives — "understory circles," neighborhood cooperatives, shared groves — can sustain the social roots of this movement. The goal is not only reforestation but reconnection: creating spaces where diverse participants share labor, story, and harvest. In these settings, therapy ceases to be a clinical intervention and becomes a collective practice of tending — of life attending to life.

To cultivate chestnuts is to affirm that healing is mutual — that human and habitat recover together, or not at all. The chestnut's return signals more than ecological resilience; it marks a turning point in consciousness, a rediscovery of belonging as the foundation of sanity, a reawakening of belonging. In planting a tree that will outlive us, we remember what time asks of us: to become ancestors, not just consumers.

In time, perhaps, the groves themselves will teach what no doctrine can: that meaning is made, not found; that strength is quiet and cumulative; that wholeness grows from attention. In the shaded dirt beneath their canopies, one might imagine a new culture taking root — one that remembers how to live with the world rather than upon it.

The way forward may not be in another invention, but in an old and patient act — to plant, to tend, and to remain long enough to witness life's quiet return.

# References

1. Centers for Disease Control and Prevention. (2024). *Suicide data and statistics.* https://www.cdc.gov/suicide/facts/data.html

2. Capaldi, C. A., Dopko, R. L., & Zelenski, J. M. (2014). The relationship between nature connectedness and happiness: A meta-analysis. *Frontiers in Psychology, 5*, Article 976. https://doi.org/10.3389/fpsyg.2014.00976

3. Rosen, L. D., et al. (2011). An empirical examination of the educational impact of text message-induced task switching in the classroom. *Educational Psychology, 31*(2), 93–109. https://doi.org/10.1080/01443410.2010.51867

4. Louv, R. (2008). *Last Child in the Woods: Saving Our Children from Nature-Deficit Disorder.* Algonquin Books

5. Bratman, G. N., Hamilton, J. P., & Daily, G. C. (2012). The impacts of nature experience on human cognitive function and mental health. *Annals of the New York Academy of Sciences, 1249*(1), 118–136. https://doi.org/10.1111/j.1749-6632.2011.06400.x

6. Jordan, M., & Hinds, J. (Eds.). (2016). *Ecotherapy: Theory, Research and Practice.* Palgrave Macmillan.

7. Gigliotti, C. M., & Jarrott, S. E. (2005). Horticultural therapy: A psychosocial intervention for older adults. *Journal of Psychosocial Nursing and Mental Health Services, 43*(9), 34–42. https://doi.org/10.3928/02793695-20050901-04

8. van der Kolk, B. A. (2014). *The Body Keeps the Score: Brain, Mind, and Body in the Healing of Trauma.* Viking.

9. Poulsen, D. V., Stigsdotter, U. K., & Davidsen, A. S. (2015). Health promotion for people with stress-related illness through nature-based therapy: Qualitative study. *Journal of Therapeutic Horticulture, 25*(1)

10. O'Brien, L., & Murray, R. (2007). Forest school and its impacts on young children: Case studies in Britain. *Urban Forestry & Urban Greening, 6*(4), 249–265. https://doi.org/10.1016/j.ufug.2007.08.003

11. Anagnostakis, S. L. (2005). The American chestnut: Its past, present, and future. *Journal of the American Chestnut Foundation, 19*(1)

12. Abram, D. (1997). *The Spell of the Sensuous: Perception and Language in a More-Than-Human World.* Vintage.

13. van Rompay, T. J. L., & Jol, T. (2016). Wild and free: Unpredictability and perceived freedom in natural versus designed environments. *Frontiers in Psychology, 7*, Article 533. https://doi.org/10.3389/fpsyg.2016.00533

14. United States Department of Veterans Affairs. (2023). *Therapeutic gardening programs for veterans: Annual Report 2023.* Office of Mental Health and Suicide Prevention, U.S. Department of Veterans Affairs.

15. Jose, S. (2009). Agroforestry for ecosystem services and environmental benefits: An overview. *Agroforestry Systems, 76*(1), 1–10. https://doi.org/10.1007/s10457-009-9229-7

# PAPER 2:

# PERENNIAL RESILIENCE

## Chestnut Agroforestry and the Regeneration of America's Soils

## Executive Summary

Soils across much of the southeastern United States are impoverished by a century of intensive annual cropping, repeated tillage, and the simplification of landscape structure. Rebuilding soil organic matter and restoring biological continuity are now central to both climate mitigation and to farm-level resilience. Perennial tree-crop systems — in particular, chestnut (*Castanea* spp.) agroforestry — offer a pragmatic, scalable pathway to reverse topsoil loss, sequester carbon, enhance water infiltration, and produce an edible, storable carbohydrate for local markets. When deployed on appropriate sites in the Piedmont and coastal plain of the Carolinas, chestnut systems can reduce sediment delivery to waterways, boost persistence of soil organic carbon, and diversify farm incomes while providing habitat and shade that moderate local climate extremes.[1]

## Why Soils Matter Now

Soil is the substrate of agriculture, the home of biological processes that sustain fertility, and a major terrestrial carbon reservoir. When soil organic matter declines, two linked problems arise: (1) the soil's ability to retain water and nutrients collapses, increasing vulnerability to drought and storm runoff; (2) previously stabilized carbon is oxidized and returned to the atmosphere, worsening climate change and creating a reinforcing feedback loop of degradation. Recent regional assessments show that Southeastern soils — particularly those on Ultisols and deeply weathered Piedmont profiles — now contain substantially less organic carbon than their pre-cultivation baselines, with measurable effects on hydrological buffering and crop resilience.[2] This trend is aggravated in eastern North Carolina, where sandy coastal-plain textures and eroded Piedmont knolls respond poorly to annual tillage and intense rainfall events.

Given those realities, an intervention is especially valuable that simultaneously (a) restores soil organic matter, (b) reduces erosion and nutrient export, and (c) generates durable on-farm economic value. Chestnut agroforestry meets all three criteria: it is a perennial system that feeds soil life year-round, intercepts and absorbs rainfall, and produces starchy nuts that can be processed and marketed regionally.

## The Agronomic Logic of Perenniality

Annual cropping systems require repeated soil disturbance to establish each year's plantings; each disturbance interrupts the root-fungal-soil food web and accelerates oxidation of stable organic fractions. Perennials, by contrast, provide continuous living roots and litter inputs, enabling the accumulation of particulate and mineral-associated organic matter in both topsoil and subsoil horizons. Meta-analyses across temperate agroforestry systems consistently find that tree integration into farmland increases soil organic carbon (SOC) relative to treeless controls, with measurable gains concentrated in the biologically active root zone.[1][3]

From a mechanistic perspective, perennial woody roots feed mycorrhizal networks whose hyphal exudates stabilize aggregates and protect organic matter from rapid decomposition. Leaf litter and fine-root turnover add continuous carbon inputs that, under low-disturbance regimes, shift the soil community toward fungal-dominated pathways associated with greater aggregate stability and longer carbon residence times.[4]

## Chestnuts: Biology, Yield Potential, and Food Value

Chestnuts occupy a distinct nutritional niche among tree nuts: unlike lipid-rich walnuts or pecans, chestnuts are starch-rich — closer in function to grains in many cuisines. Their carbohydrate-dominant kernels are low in fat and can be roasted, boiled, or milled into flour — making them an adaptable local staple for breads, porridges, and processed goods that fit gluten-free and whole-food markets.[5]

Modern chestnut plantings use hybrids (often Chinese × American or improved cultivars) that deliver earlier bearing and improved disease resilience compared with unselected seedling stands. Under suitable site conditions and with proper management, mature chestnut plantings can yield 2,000–4,000 lb. per acre of in-shell nuts — a meaningful calorie and income stream for family-scale farms.[13][14]

## Carbon, Water, and Soil: What Evidence Shows

Extensive research has been done with a broad range of studies and analyses of how chestnut cultivation affects the land. In general, this approach compares favorably with other agricultural systems in place throughout the Southeast. Three categories worth touching on here are Soil Organic Carbon gains, water flow and erosion issues, and a carbon-capture perspective.

### Soil Organic Carbon Gains in Temperate Agroforestry
Observational and meta-analytic work shows that temperate agroforestry systems can increase SOC relative to adjacent cropland within decades.[137]

### Hydrology and Erosion Control
Chestnut plantings intercept rainfall and decelerate overland flow, reducing sheet erosion and suspended sediment delivery to streams — an outcome especially important for watersheds draining to North Carolina's sensitive estuaries.[289]

### Carbon Accounting — Above and Below Ground
Chestnut systems sequester carbon both in woody biomass and in the soil. Recent modeling demonstrates that combined above- and below-ground sequestration can yield significant and even multi-ton carbon gains per acre over decades, depending on tree density and site productivity.[137]

## Regional Relevance: Eastern North Carolina and the Carolinas

The eastern and central Carolinas blend several landform types — sandy coastal plain, Sandhills, and clay-rich Piedmont uplands — each with specific soil vulnerabilities. In the coastal plain, coarse-textured profiles drain quickly and are prone to nutrient leaching and salt intrusion as sea-level rise advances. In the Piedmont, long histories of cultivation have exposed red subsoils high in iron and clay but low in organic matter and structure.[2 9]

Chestnuts are well adapted to these environments in several ways: deep fibrous roots that fracture compacted layers, tolerance to a range of soil textures, and litter that contributes labile organic matter. When integrated into riparian buffers and contour plantings, trees like chestnuts can reduce sediment transport into the Neuse, Tar-Pamlico, and Cape Fear Basins — watersheds where nutrient loads and turbidity are persistent concerns.[2 8 10]

Finally, the region's foodways provide cultural openings for chestnuts: historic Appalachian and Southern culinary traditions include chestnut-based dishes, creating potential local demand when combined with value-added processing.[13 14]

## Implementation Pathways

Scaling chestnut agroforestry involves four interlinked domains: science (breeding and monitoring), finance (business models and incentives), infrastructure (nursery and processing capacity), and culture (markets and community adoption).[11 12]

### 1. Research and Technical Support
Land-grant institutions and USDA programs can host multi-site trials monitoring SOC beneath chestnut systems across coastal and Piedmont soils.[12]

### 2. Financial Incentives and Risk Management
Public programs can adapt to perennial realities by offering multi-year cost-share and deferred-repayment loans targeted to food-bearing perennials.[12]

### 3. Infrastructure and Value Chains
Cooperative shelling/drying facilities can reduce per-farm capital barriers and enable aggregation for regional processors.[13 14]

### 4. Outreach and Cultural Integration
Demonstration orchards and community plantings can provide visible models, while culinary partnerships generate cultural momentum.[13 14]

## Risks, Constraints, and Mitigation

Chestnut agroforestry is not universal. Constraints include unsuitable drainage in some locations, the time lag to production, and pest or disease pressures (notably chestnut blight). These are manageable through common-sense site planning, cultivar selection, genetic diversity, and integrated pest management.[11][15]

## Policy Recommendations (Summary)

1. Authorize and fund perennial food-tree establishment within federal and state conservation programs.[12]
2. Fund multi-site cultivar and soil-monitoring trials via land-grant universities.[12]
3. Support rural cooperative processing infrastructure.[13][14]
4. Create establishment finance tools and carbon-accounting protocols for chestnut systems.[12]
5. Invest in outreach and culinary partnerships to build public familiarity.[13][14]

## Conclusion

Chestnut agroforestry offers a rare synthesis of ecological repair and human provisioning. It addresses the urgent need to rebuild soil organic matter, buffer hydrology, sequester carbon, and restore productive diversity — all while producing an edible, culturally resonant staple that local communities can process together and eat.[15]

## References

1. De Stefano A, Jacobson MG. 2018. Soil carbon sequestration in agroforestry systems: a meta-analysis. *Agrofor Syst.* 92(2):285–299. Available from: https://doi.org/10.1007/s10457-017-0147-9
2. US Global Change Research Program. 2023. Chapter 22: The Southeast. In: *Fifth National Climate Assessment.* Washington (DC): US Government Publishing Office. Available from: https://nca2023.globalchange.gov/chapter/22/
3. Beillouin D, Corbeels M, Cardinael R, et al. 2023. A global meta-analysis of soil organic carbon in the Anthropocene. *Nat Commun.* 14:3700. Available from: https://doi.org/10.1038/s41467-023-39338-z
4. Franzluebbers AJ. 2023. Root-zone enrichment of soil-test biological activity and particulate organic carbon and nitrogen under conventional and conservation land management. *Soil Sci Soc Am J.* 87:1431–1443. Available from: https://doi.org/10.1002/saj2.20574
5. American Chestnut Foundation. 2024. Restoration and breeding resources. Asheville (NC): The American Chestnut Foundation. Available from: https://www.tacf.org

6.  Eddy WC, Yang WH. 2022. Improvements in soil health and soil carbon sequestration by an agroforestry for food production system. *Agric Ecosyst Environ.* 333:107945. Available from: https://doi.org/10.1016/j.agee.2022.107945

7.  Montagnini F, Nair PKR. 2004. Carbon sequestration: an underexploited environmental benefit of agroforestry systems. *Agrofor Syst.* 61–62:281–295. Available from: https://doi.org/10.1023/B:AGFO.0000029005.92691.79

8.  Veldkamp E, Schmidt M, Markwitz C, et al. 2023. Multifunctionality of temperate alley-cropping agroforestry outperforms open cropland and grassland. *Commun Earth Environ.* 4:20. Available from: https://doi.org/10.1038/s43247-023-00680-1

9.  US Global Change Research Program. 2023. Southeastern coastal and Piedmont soil degradation indicators. In: *Fifth National Climate Assessment,* Chapter 22. Washington (DC): US Government Publishing Office.

10. Franzluebbers AJ, Langdale GW. 2021. Soil organic carbon and nitrogen fractionation in agricultural systems under conservation management. *Soil Tillage Res.* 215:105231. Available from: https://doi.org/10.1016/j.still.2021.105231

11. American Chestnut Foundation. 2024. Regional adaptation and blight resistance trials. Asheville (NC): The American Chestnut Foundation. Available from: https://www.tacf.org

12. US Global Change Research Program. 2023. Economic transitions and agricultural adaptation in the Southeast (NCA5 Technical Annex). Washington (DC): US Government Publishing Office.

13. Gold MA, Cernusca MM, Godsey LD. 2005. Chestnut market report. Columbia (MO): University of Missouri Center for Agroforestry. Available from: https://centerforagroforestry.org

14. Savanna Institute. 2024. Chestnut industry implementation plan for the Midwest and Eastern US. Madison (WI): Savanna Institute. Available from: https://www.savannainstitute.org

15. American Chestnut Foundation. 2024. Restoration progress report: breeding for resistance and regional adaptation. Asheville (NC): The American Chestnut Foundation. Available from: https://www.tacf.org

PAPER 3:

# ROOTED RENEWAL

## Chestnuts and the Rebuilding of Rural America

## Executive Summary

Rural communities across the United States — and especially in the Carolinas — face converging economic, social, and ecological strains. Decades of farm consolidation, dependence on annual monocultures, and market centralization have left many family farms economically precarious and local food systems brittle. Chestnut cultivation (*Castanea* spp.), practiced at scale as a perennial agroforestry crop, offers an integrative alternative: a nutritious, storable starchy food; a low-input perennial that rebuilds soil and stores carbon; and a generational enterprise that can reconnect families and neighbors to a place-based economy and culture.

This white paper argues that a coordinated public–private effort to expand chestnut agroforestry — combining support for growers, investment in mid-scale processing, and extension research on regionally adapted cultivars (including blight-resistant hybrids) — can deliver simultaneous benefits for rural livelihoods, local food security, and ecological restoration.

## Background: How the Crisis Shows Up in the Carolinas

Since the mid-twentieth century, the U.S. has seen a steady decline in the number of farms and an ongoing concentration of acreage in larger operations. After peaking at roughly 6.8 million farms in the 1930s, farm numbers have dropped to well under two million in recent years.[1] These national dynamics are visible in North Carolina's coastal plain, Sandhills, and Piedmont, where small diversified farms were gradually replaced by commodity row crops and vertically integrated livestock operations; the result has been a concentration of value upstream while costs and environmental burdens accumulate locally.[2]

Corn and soy dominate U.S. crop acreage. In many counties of the Carolinas, row crops and industrial livestock production have placed persistent pressure on soils and watersheds. Repeated annual tillage, heavy synthetic fertilizer use, and simplified crop rotations have reduced organic matter and increased runoff and erosion on both clay-rich Piedmont soils and sandy coastal plain loams.[3] On a human level, with problems like restricted access to land for new entrants and reduced local civic capacity, rural communities show measurable mental health disparities. Economic precarity and the erosion of place-based livelihoods have measurable social impacts: population aging and decline in some rural towns, rising indicators of distress.[4]

## Chestnut Agroforestry: The Science and Suitability for the Carolinas

Chestnuts are fast-maturing relative to many forest trees, can be highly productive as orchard crops, and adapt to a range of temperate soils. Modern cultivar programs (notably grafted Chinese chestnut cultivars and American × Chinese hybrids such as the Eaton and the Dunstan) combine vigor, nut quality, and improved disease tolerance.[5] Establishment commonly requires 4–7 years before full bearing, though farmers may see lower yields earlier from young trees.[6] Mature, well-managed chestnut orchards can produce hundreds to thousands of pounds per acre (extension estimates commonly cite ranges around 1,000–3,000 lb/acre depending on cultivar and management).[6]

Because chestnuts are perennials with no annual tillage needs, their long-term input profile is lower than those of many annual commodity rotations. Chestnuts are carbohydrate-rich relative to other tree nuts, providing a starchy, gluten-free flour option and a versatile culinary ingredient.[7]

## Pathways to Local Economic Renewal

Chestnuts create layered revenue possibilities: fresh and processed nut sales, chestnut flour and value-added products for regional bakeries and specialty food markets, nursery stock, and agritourism. Regional market studies and grower surveys historically find that consumer demand outpaces domestic supply; in many areas producers sell out quickly.[8] Investments in shared processing (shelling, drying, cold storage) and cooperative marketing enable small orchards to access broader markets without large capital outlays.[9] Cooperative and producer associations can lower barriers for small growers by sharing equipment and pursuing joint branding.[10]

## Ecological Benefits: Soil, Carbon, and Landscape Resilience

Tree systems including chestnuts stabilize surface soils with permanent root networks and reduce erosion compared with continuous annual tillage. Deep litter layers contribute organic matter over time and support soil aggregation and microbial communities.[11] Perennial woody biomass stores carbon aboveground and belowground; reviews find that agroforestry systems can deliver meaningful carbon sequestration per hectare while provisioning food.[12] Chestnut groves provide habitat structure, reduce runoff peaks, and create microclimates beneficial to understory crops or livestock.

## Social and Cultural Renewal

A perennial food culture encourages patience, reciprocal labor, and shared stewardship. Chestnut harvests, processing days, and festivals can reanimate local economies and restore ritual markers of seasonality.[13] Evidence links nature exposure and participation in nature-based programs to reduced stress, improved mood, and better cognitive outcomes; chestnut cultivation fits naturally within such therapeutic and vocational frameworks.[14]

## A Practical Policy Framework

To scale chestnut agroforestry in ways that favor family-based renewal, policymakers and civic leaders should pursue coordinated enabling actions:

A. Align conservation payments with perennial systems.[15]
B. Bridge establishment finance using low-interest loans.[16]
C. Invest in mid-scale processing and regional value chains.[17]
D. Scale extension and cultivar adaptation research.[18]
F. Support education, apprenticeship, and veteran pathways.[19]

## Planting for Generations

Chestnuts are both pragmatic and symbolic: a practical perennial starch with proven yields and real market demand with future potential, and a living emblem of stewardship that rewards multi-generational thinking. In the Carolinas, where soils, culture, and climate converge, chestnut agroforestry can help restore ecological function, provide diversified family incomes, and revive place-centered community life. With thoughtful policy alignment, targeted investment, and sustained research support, a coordinated chestnut revival could help re-root rural America.

## References

1. USDA National Agricultural Statistics Service (USDA NASS). 2024. *2022 census of agriculture: United States summary and state data.* Washington (DC): U.S. Department of Agriculture. Available from: https://www.nass.usda.gov/Publications/AgCensus/2022/index.php
2. USDA Economic Research Service (USDA ERS). 2023. *Farm household income and characteristics.* Washington (DC): U.S. Department of Agriculture. Available from: https://www.ers.usda.gov/data-products/farm-household-income-and-characteristics
3. U.S. Geological Survey (USGS). 2023. *Cropland data layer.* Washington (DC): U.S. Department of the Interior. Available from: https://nassgeodata.gmu.edu/CropScape
4. Morales DA, Young M, McIntosh WL, Eagan R, Martinez L. 2020. Rural mental health disparities in the United States: current challenges and opportunities. *Int J Environ Res Public Health.* 17(24):9225. https://doi.org/10.3390/ijerph17249225
5. Revord RS. 2022. *Growing and marketing Chinese chestnuts.* Columbia (MO): University of Missouri Center for Agroforestry. Available from: https://centerforagroforestry.org
6. University of Missouri Center for Agroforestry (UMCA). 2023. *Chestnut cultivar trial summaries, 2020–2023.* Columbia (MO): UMCA. Available from: https://centerforagroforestry.org/wp-content/uploads/2023/07/Cultivar_Trial_Summary_2020_2023.pdf
7. Santos MJ, Barros L, Martins N, Silva S, Ferreira ICFR. 2022. Sweet chestnut (*Castanea sativa* Mill.) nutritional and antioxidant properties: a comprehensive study. *Foods.* 11(21):3335. https://doi.org/10.3390/foods11213335
8. Gold MA, Cernusca MM, Godsey LD. 2005. *Chestnut market report.* Columbia (MO): University of Missouri Center for Agroforestry. Available from: https://centerforagroforestry.org/wp-content/uploads/2016/05/ChestnutMarketReport05.pdf
9. The American Chestnut Foundation (TACF). 2023. *Restoration science program overview.* Asheville (NC): TACF. Available from: https://www.acf.org/science
10. USDA Rural Development (USDA RD). 2024. *Value-added producer grants (VAPG) program.* Washington (DC): U.S. Department of Agriculture. Available from: https://www.rd.usda.gov/programs-services/business-programs/value-added-producer-grants

11. Daniels RB. 2019. *Soil erosion in the Southern Piedmont.* Raleigh (NC): North Carolina Cooperative Extension. Available from: https://www.ncagr.gov/soil/erosion
12. Castle SE, Corstanje R, Quinn N, Hannah MA. 2022. Quantifying the contribution of agroforestry to climate-change mitigation in temperate regions: a systematic map. *Environ Evid.* 11:15. https://doi.org/10.1186/s13750-022-00280-y
13. University of Missouri Center for Agroforestry (UMCA). 2023. *Extension and outreach: demonstrations, resources, and grower education.* Columbia (MO): UMCA. Available from: https://centerforagroforestry.org/extension-outreach
14. Clay R. 2023. Ecotherapy and environmental restoration. *Monitor on Psychology.* 54(6):48–53. Available from: https://www.apa.org/monitor/2023/06/cover-ecotherapy
15. USDA Natural Resources Conservation Service (USDA NRCS). 2023. *Conservation stewardship program handbook.* Washington (DC): U.S. Department of Agriculture. Available from: https://www.nrcs.usda.gov/resources/guides-and-instructions/conservation-stewardship-program-handbook
16. USDA Farm Service Agency (USDA FSA). 2023. *Microloan and beginning farmer program documentation.* Washington (DC): U.S. Department of Agriculture. Available from: https://www.fsa.usda.gov/programs-and-services/farm-loan-programs/microloans/index
17. USDA Rural Development (USDA RD). 2023. *Examples of VAPG and processing grants.* Washington (DC): U.S. Department of Agriculture. Available from: https://www.rd.usda.gov/programs-services/value-added-producer-grants
18. The American Chestnut Foundation (TACF). 2023. *Science & research update: breeding, trials, and disease resistance.* Asheville (NC): TACF. Available from: https://www.acf.org/wp-content/uploads/2023/09/TACF-2023-Science-Update.pdf
19. U.S. Department of Veterans Affairs (VA). 2023. *Agriculture and nature-based therapy pilot programs.* Washington (DC): U.S. Department of Veterans Affairs. Available from: https://www.mentalhealth.va.gov/

ESSAY:

# BEYOND PINE

## The Long-Term Economics and Ecology of Chestnut Orchards versus Southern Pine Plantations

*...slower to begin, but enduring for generations; humbler in initial return, yet ultimately far more regenerative in wealth, soil, and meaning....*

**Across much of** the southeastern United States, the rural horizon is drawn by straight lines of pine. Loblolly and slash plantations march in regimented grids across the Sandhills and uplands, their needles whispering a dry hymn to the logic of industrial forestry. For decades this model has been the default means of "reforesting" cutover land: plant fast-growing conifers, harvest at thirty years, repeat. It is a formula optimized for pulp and timber markets, a rotation economy that prizes short-term yield and standardized management.

But another perennial system is quietly re-emerging—one whose lineage once defined the eastern forest economy. The chestnut orchard, blending tree crops with human food production, offers a radically different economic rhythm: slower to begin, but enduring for generations; humbler in initial return, yet ultimately far more regenerative in wealth, soil, and meaning. When compared side by side, pine plantations and chestnut orchards represent two distinct cultural and ecological philosophies of land use—two divergent futures for rural landscapes and those who tend them.

## Lifespan and Temporal Economics

The pine plantation is built on the rotation: a 25–35-year arc from planting to harvest, when the stand is clear-cut and the cycle begins anew. Its logic is one of liquidation and re-establishment. Each cohort of trees is a discrete investment; capital and soil carbon are both reset at each harvest.

Chestnuts, by contrast, inhabit time differently. Once established, a chestnut orchard matures gradually and remains productive for a century or more. Hybrid American lines typically begin to bear lightly around year eight, reach commercial production by year twelve, and often sustain annual yields for many human generations. Their economic rhythm is not one of periodic liquidation, but of continual, renewable yield—an annuity rather than a bond that must be cashed out.

When discounted over the long term, this temporal distinction transforms the financial calculus. A loblolly stand yielding $1,500 per acre every 30 years can generate an internal rate of return of roughly 4–6%—serviceable, but dependent on low land costs, cheap labor, and steady pulp demand. A chestnut system that nets $3,000–$5,000 per acre annually at maturity, even after higher establishment and maintenance costs, can sustain returns in the 12–15% range. More importantly, its productive asset continues indefinitely: every additional decade compounds value without replanting or re-disturbing the soil. Over a 100-year horizon, pine is a succession of harvests; chestnut is a living endowment.

## Soil and Ecological Function

From a distance, both pines and chestnuts green the land, sequester carbon, and offer wildlife shelter. Yet their effects on the soil diverge sharply beneath the litter layer. Pine needles acidify and simplify the forest floor, supporting limited fungal diversity and slowing decomposition. The heavy equipment required for harvest compacts subsoils, increasing runoff and reducing infiltration. Carbon accumulation under pine stands is modest and often offset by disturbance losses at clear-cutting. In other words, the physical ground of the property loses its natural value over time.

Chestnuts, by contrast, enrich the soil with calcium-rich litter, promoting a thriving web of mycorrhizae and decomposers. Their wide canopies admit dappled light that nurtures an understory of perennial grasses, forbs, and fungi. In integrated alley systems, farmers can graze livestock or cultivate mushrooms and herbs without degrading soil structure. Long-term studies show 20–50% gains in soil organic carbon under well-managed nut agroforestry within a decade—a living counterbalance to the extractive pulse of pine rotations. In a chestnut orchard, the land's fertility naturally grows over time.

Hydrologically, chestnut systems behave more like natural forests: deep rooting increases infiltration and stabilizes water tables, reducing erosion and nutrient loss. Their leaf litter buffers pH and returns minerals to the topsoil, sustaining fertility without synthetic input. In short, the chestnut orchard regenerates the foundation that the pine plantation merely occupies.

## Market Structure and Value Chains

The pine industry is a triumph of scale and standardization. Mechanized planting, fertilization, thinning, and clear-cutting have reduced costs to the bare minimum. But this efficiency hides fragility: revenues hinge on global pulp and sawtimber markets, which fluctuate with construction cycles and trade policy. The small landowner of a pine plantation remains a price-taker, dependent on distant mills and brokers.

*The small landowner of a pine plantation remains a price-taker, dependent on distant mills and brokers.*

Chestnuts operate in a younger, more diversified market space. Demand for gluten-free flour, plant-based proteins, and perennial agroforestry crops has surged, while domestic supply remains limited. Wholesale prices of $1.50–$2.50 per pound, and retail prices of $3–$4, are common. Processed products—flour, puree, roasted nuts—capture higher margins still. Cooperative marketing models can return 70–80% of sale value to growers, particularly where processing and branding remain local.

Unlike timber, nut production provides **annual income** after establishment, allowing for reinvestment, labor stability, and a human relationship with the crop that endures. The orchardist is not waiting decades for a lump-sum harvest; they are harvesting each season, refining quality, and building regional identity. This structure turns farming from speculative cycle to steady livelihood.

## Risk and Resilience

Pine is a high-volume, low-margin commodity exposed to market, weather, and fire risk. A single hurricane or price slump can erase a decade of compounding growth. Insurance mechanisms exist, but they favor large corporate owners who can pool thousands of acres.

Chestnut systems distribute risk differently. Yields fluctuate with weather and pollination, but total loss is rare. The trees themselves, once mature, withstand drought and moderate fire, and can coppice from the base if damaged, unlike pines. Furthermore, multiple income streams—fresh nuts, processed foods, agrotourism, nursery operations, even selective timber harvest—diversify exposure. The result is a more **resilient revenue curve**, less volatile than the boom-and-bust of pulp market cycles.

For the state or region, this stability translates into predictable rural income and reduced environmental liability. Where pine landscapes burn, chestnut landscapes buffer and feed.

## Social and Cultural Dimensions

The industrial pine model suits absentee ownership: large tracts managed remotely, few jobs per acre, profits exported to distant corporations. It reinforces a geography of extraction—wealth flowing out of rural counties as raw material, leaving little cultural residue behind.

Chestnut orchards, on the other hand, lend themselves to local stewardship. They fit the scale of family farms, veterans' programs, educational institutions, and cooperatives. Because the trees live a century and longer, they root families and communities in a shared temporal horizon. The act of tending them becomes intergenerational—a lived inheritance.

## Shared Benefits

To be fair, pine plantations are not without merit. They sequester carbon, protect eroding soils compared to bare cropland, and can provide transitional cover for wildlife. Both systems, when managed thoughtfully, participate in the global work of reforestation and carbon sequestration.

Indeed, a hybrid landscape—where chestnut orchards are interspersed with long-rotation pine and mixed hardwood corridors—could deliver the best of both: the carbon density of softwoods, the fertility and human value of nut agroforestry. The question is not pine *or* chestnut, but which system should anchor the next century's working lands.

## Profitability Across Time

Consider two hypothetical five-acre parcels, side by side in the North Carolina Sandhills. One is planted to loblolly pine, the other to chestnut. The pine stand may cost about $2,500 to establish and yield $7,500 after thirty years—a modest return that, after discounting, barely doubles the original investment. The chestnut orchard can cost up to $19,000 to plant and maintain but begins generating $15,000–$25,000 annually from year twelve onward. By year twenty, it has not only repaid its establishment cost but has produced cumulative profits several times greater than the pine parcel's lifetime value.

*The pine model monetizes depletion; the chestnut model monetizes renewal.*

Extend the horizon to fifty years, and the divergence becomes profound: the pine land has undergone two harvest cycles, leaving compacted soils and modest net income; the chestnut land continues to bear food, build carbon, and support livelihoods without replanting. Its productive asset has *appreciated* with time rather than depreciated with harvest.

This is not simply a difference in rate of return. It is a difference in what "return" means. The pine model monetizes depletion; the chestnut model monetizes renewal.

## Toward a Perennial Economy

At the policy level, the contrast invites rethinking of incentives. For decades, public cost-share programs and timber tax structures have favored pine: low establishment grants, rapid write-offs, and clear definitions of "forest products." Chestnut and other agroforestry crops fall between categories—neither conventional agriculture nor recognized timber—leaving growers without equivalent support.

Correcting this imbalance would require little more than adjusting existing frameworks: extending reforestation cost-shares to nut agroforestry, offering low-interest loans through state development banks, and funding regional processing cooperatives. The long-term fiscal payoff—steady rural employment, enhanced water quality, carbon credits, and reduced wildfire risk—would far exceed the modest public investment.

Such policy realignment would also signal a deeper cultural shift: from short-rotation extraction to long-rotation regeneration; from export of raw material to cultivation of value at home.

## The Broader Ledger

In the strict ledger of finance, pine yields a known quantity at known intervals. In the broader ledger of the land, it often runs a deficit—of nutrients, biodiversity, and local agency. Chestnut systems, though slower to mature, accumulate compound interest in three important ways: ecological, economic, and human.

Over a century, a pine landscape cycles through clear-cuts and regrowth, oscillating between plenty and emptiness. A chestnut landscape, once established, becomes a permanent structure of fertility—a food forest that pays dividends every autumn. In a changing, unstable climate, such continuity is its own form of wealth.

## Conclusion: Two Models of Permanence

Both pine and chestnut promise permanence, but of different kinds. Pine offers the permanence of a system: industrial, replicable, and uniform. Chestnut offers the permanence of relationship: ecological, cultural, and intergenerational.

If the aim of rural development is to generate not only profit but *place*, then chestnut agroforestry stands as the more enduring investment. Its returns accrue in living soil, in annual harvests, in work that restores rather than exhausts. It is, in economic and moral terms alike, the better compounder of interest.

The question, then, is not whether we can afford to replace pine with chestnut, but whether we can afford **not** to—when the latter builds the kind of wealth that lasts a century and longer.

ESSAY:

# THE ROMAN CHESTNUT

How an Empire Rooted a Foreign Tree Across the Old World

## Origins: From the Edge of Empire

This history lesson begins long before the Roman legions crossed the Alps. Already, the chestnut tree grew wild in the mountainous margins of the eastern Mediterranean. *Castanea sativa*, the sweet chestnut, was native not to Gaul or Hispania but to the humid uplands of Anatolia, the Caucasus, and parts of Greece and southern Italy. There, among mixed oak and beech forests, people gathered its nuts for millennia. By the classical Greek period, it was already known as *kástanon*, a tree associated with Thessaly and Pontus, regions famed for their fertile slopes and long cultural exchange with Persia.

The Greeks valued the chestnut as both food and medicine. Dioscorides and Theophrastus described its virtues, while farmers learned to graft superior varieties, selecting for larger and sweeter nuts. Yet its cultivation remained local, an eastern Mediterranean specialty—one among many fruits in the diversified orchards of antiquity. The chestnut's transformation from regional food to continental staple awaited a people with roads, armies, and an appetite for permanence.

## Rome's Agricultural Ambition

The Romans inherited and expanded the Greek horticultural tradition but directed it toward imperial purpose. Their genius was not invention but integration: taking a species, a technology, or a crop and deploying it across climates, markets, and provinces. The chestnut, with its durable, storable nut and long-lived timber, fit perfectly into this system.

Writers like Virgil, Columella, and Pliny the Elder praised the chestnut as a highland counterpart to the olive—a tree comfortable in marginal soils that produced both food and wood. Columella recommended grafting and spacing methods that mirror modern orchard design. Chestnuts fed peasants and soldiers alike: boiled, roasted, or ground into meal. Unlike grain, they could be harvested even from steep slopes unsuitable for plowing, turning neglected terrain into productive landscape.

As the empire spread, so did its tree crops. The legions brought not only law and roads but seeds and scions. Military garrisons planted orchards near fortresses to ensure local provisioning. Settlers from Italy established villas that replicated the home landscapes of Campania and Etruria, chestnuts included. From these nuclei the species radiated outward—down valleys, along trade routes, and across mountain frontiers.

## Naturalization: From Cultivated Grove to Forest Citizen

By the first centuries of the Common Era, chestnuts had taken root far beyond their ancestral range. In Gaul, along the Pyrenees and Massif Central, they flourished in volcanic soils. In Hispania and Lusitania they climbed the Atlantic slopes, displacing oaks in certain niches. Even in the damp hills of Britannia, Roman estates left pollen traces of chestnut groves where none had grown before.

Once planted, chestnuts proved hardy and fecund. Their nuts, carried by animals or washed down streams, germinated freely. Over generations the line between orchard and forest blurred. Abandoned villas left behind groves that reverted to semi-wild stands. Local people gathered nuts, coppiced stems, and developed landraces adapted to regional microclimates.

By the early Middle Ages, chestnuts were no longer a foreign species but a familiar neighbor. Genetic studies show remarkable regional differentiation—proof of long residence and human selection. The tree that Rome had exported as an imperial crop had become a citizen of countless local ecologies, shaped by climate, culture, and time.

## The Medieval Bread Tree

In the centuries after Rome's fall, monasteries became stewards of chestnut groves, maintaining grafting knowledge and developing new uses for the wood and tannins. The tree's endurance through political chaos made it a symbol of stability.

Across the Apennines, the Cévennes, the Basque Country, and Corsica, chestnuts sustained entire mountain economies. The nuts were dried in stone kilns and ground into flour—*farina dolce*—that served as staple food through winters when grain failed. In some regions the chestnut was called *l'arbre à pain*, the bread tree, its yield literally feeding villages for centuries.

Medieval coppice systems allowed repeated harvest of poles for fencing, fuel, and construction without killing the tree. The result was an agroforestry mosaic of extraordinary longevity: some stands in Italy and France trace their genetic lineage back over a thousand years. Here, the chestnut had completed its metamorphosis—from imported orchard tree to keystone of local subsistence and identity.

## Ecology and the Meaning of "Native"

Two millennia later, it is difficult to speak of the chestnut in Europe as anything but native. It shelters birds and mammals, hosts complex fungal guilds, and defines the appearance of entire landscapes. Its pollen lies layered in peat cores as an unbroken record of habitation.

And yet, strictly speaking, it is an introduced species. The Roman hand that planted it is long gone, but its ecological legacy remains, blurred by time and assimilation. This raises an important ecological and philosophical question: at what point does a foreign organism, once established and integrated, become part of a place?

The European chestnut suggests that nativeness is not a static category but a temporal process—a dialogue between species and setting. Given enough centuries of cohabitation, relationships emerge, dependencies form, and the boundaries of origin fade. What was once foreign becomes at home and in time becomes wholly naturalized. The chestnut's story reminds us that belonging can be built, not just inherited.

## Empires Fade, Trees Remain

The Roman Empire fractured, its aqueducts and walls crumbled, and yet its arboreal emissaries lived on. The chestnut became a quiet continuity across political ruptures—a biological infrastructure more enduring than stone. In an age when borders shifted and tongues changed, the chestnut groves anchored rural life in an unbroken rhythm of autumn harvests.

To walk through the terraced groves of Tuscany or the Cévennes today is to step into a living archive of the Roman world's ecological reach. Each massive, gnarled trunk is a monument not of conquest but of cultivation. What began as a tool of imperial provisioning has become a shared inheritance of continents.

## Epilogue: The Return of the Chestnut

There is a certain symmetry, almost poetic, in the chestnut's modern story. Just as Rome carried the species westward two thousand years ago, we now look to reintroduce it eastward and westward again—into landscapes from which its American cousin was lost. The chestnut blight of the early twentieth century felled billions of trees and erased a cornerstone of North America's forest culture. Yet the impulse to restore it—to graft resilience onto memory—echoes the same human instinct that once spread it across the Empire: the desire to root sustenance and beauty in living wood.

The Roman diffusion of the chestnut teaches several lessons for modern restoration. First, that trees move not only with climate but with culture; they follow the paths of human care and exchange. Second, that ecosystems are not frozen tableaux but evolving partnerships capable of absorbing new members. And finally, that acts of planting can ripple through millennia, reshaping both landscape and identity for the better.

In reestablishing chestnut in American soils—through hybrid breeding, agroforestry, and community planting—we can participate in a very old tradition: the renewal of a tree that binds food, shelter, and meaning. Like the Romans, we plant not only for ourselves but for a world we will never see mature.

And if history is any guide, those who come after us may scarcely remember when the chestnut was considered foreign. They will walk beneath its shade and call it native, as if it had always belonged.

A PRACTICAL SKETCH:


## ORCHARD STARTUP EXAMPLE

This is a basic profile of a moderate-density (25 ft. average spacing) high-quality chestnut orchard with ~350 trees total, using top premium Dunstan/Eaton-type seedling stock. The orchard is 5 acres. The total establishment cost is roughly $19,000 up front (about $3,800/acre). Annual maintenance averages $3,000 across the block.

We project a 15-year horizon for this model, ramping up to full bearing by year 8, with mature yields around 2,000 lb./acre (10,000 lb. total). Cooperative marketing and processing fees are pegged at 25%.

For simplicity and caution, this example's finances are based only on bulk sales of raw chestnuts and long-term low-maintenance operations. Bear in mind that this makes it a bare minimum profile in terms of revenue (not containing numbers for value-added produce, agritourism, or other potential income streams).

## Financial projections

| Case | Price/Yield assumption | Breakeven (discounted) | NPV @ 5% | IRR |
|------|------------------------|------------------------|----------|-----|
| Best | $2.50 / lb, 2,400 lb/acre | ~Year 9 | ≈ $63 k | ~19 % |
| Base | $2.00 / lb, 2,000 lb/acre | ~Year 11 | ≈ $31 k | ~14 % |
| Conservative | $1.50 / lb, 1,600 lb/acre | ~Year 14 (barely positive) | ≈ $2–5 k | ~6 % |

- Net Present Value (NPV) chart

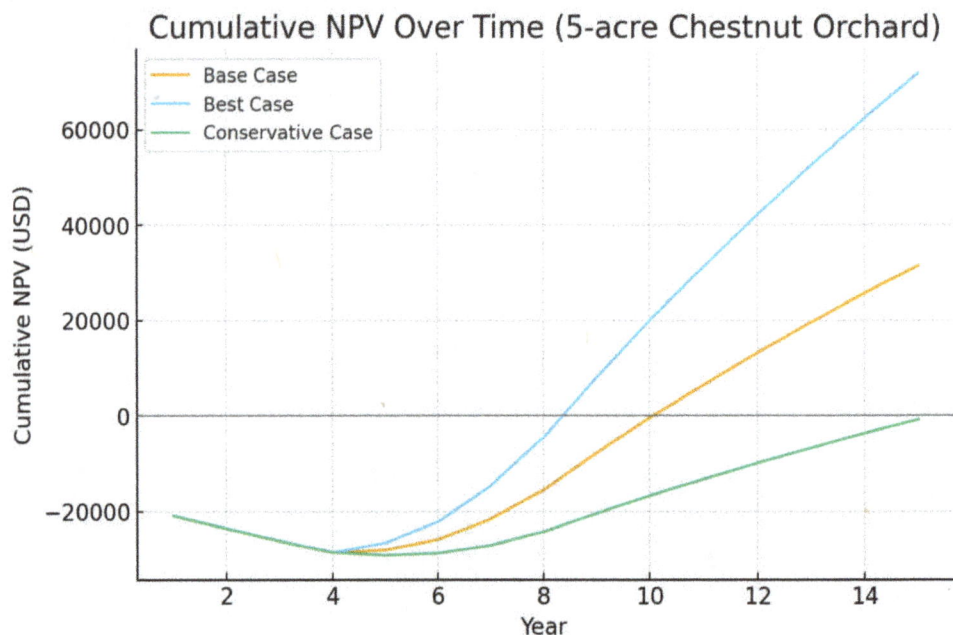

Cumulative NPV Over Time (5-acre Chestnut Orchard)

## Data Interpretation

- The orchard **operates at a loss for roughly the first eight years**, which is normal for long-lived nut trees.
- Profitability then accelerates sharply, with **positive annual cash flow after year 8** and **breakeven NPV by years 10–11** under realistic pricing.
- Even at conservative assumptions, the project remains near break-even — meaning relatively low downside risk compared to many perennial crops.

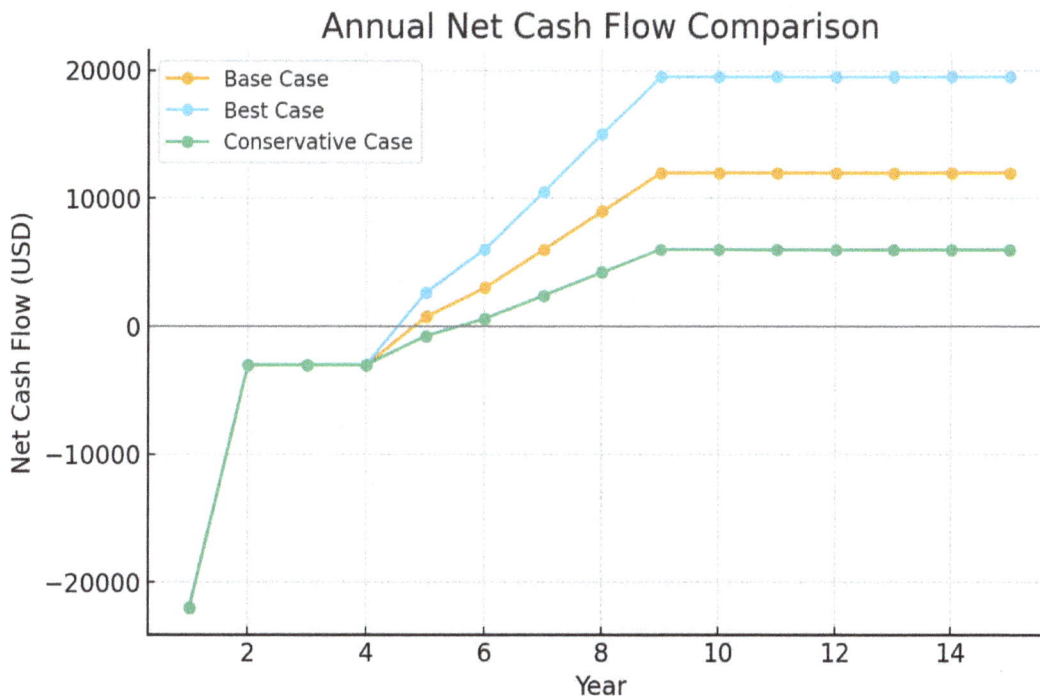

Annual Net Cash Flow Comparison

## Strategic implications

1. **Working capital & patience**
   You'll need about $25,000 liquidity (including maintenance through the establishment phase) before returns begin. Access to low-interest financing, cost-share programs, or grant support for the first 8 years would smooth the path.

2. **Cooperative leverage**
   Since cooperative fees are the largest single deduction, developing local or shared processing capacity that returns even 10% more to growers significantly boosts IRR (adds 2–3 points).

3. **Diversification & cash-flow bridges**
   Integrating intercrops or short-rotation enterprises (mushrooms, poultry, or vegetables in alleys)

can cover maintenance costs and shorten effective breakeven by 2–3 years. Further along, more processed products such as chestnut flour etc. can also boost cash flow.

4. **Market positioning**

   The difference between $1.50 and $2.50 / lb. retail price essentially doubles long-term returns. Layered operations such as direct marketing, branded value-added products, nursery business, and agritourism can make or break profitability.

5. **Resilience**

   Chestnuts show strong downside protection: even under conservative yields and low prices, you recover your investment and maintain asset value (trees and soil carbon). That's rare among specialty crops.

POLICY BRIEF:

# CHESTNUT AGROFORESTRY

A North Carolina Model

for Rural Renewal, Soil Regeneration, and Community Healing

## The Opportunity

Chestnut-based agroforestry is a *proven, perennial solution* that advances three urgent state priorities:

- **Rural Economic Revitalization** — creating year-round farm income, small-scale processing jobs, and new cooperative enterprises.
- **Soil and Water Regeneration** — restoring organic soil richness, stabilizing hydrology, and reversing erosion on degraded cropland.
- **Community Health and Belonging** — reconnecting people to land stewardship and collective purpose through long-term cultivation.

Together, these form a model of lasting resilience — integrating economic, ecological, and social renewal.

---

## Evidence Base (from The DeepRichDirt Project white papers)

- *Branches of Healing* (2025) — Documents how agroforestry programs support mental health, veteran reintegration, and community cohesion through therapeutic horticulture and collective stewardship.
- *Perennial Resilience* (2025) — Synthesizes research showing chestnut systems increase soil organic carbon by 20–50% within a decade, while reducing erosion and improving water infiltration up to 40%.
- *Rooted Renewal* (2025) — Demonstrates how processing cooperatives and regional value chains can keep 70–80% of profits local, creating rural multiplier effects of 2–3×.

---

## Policy Levers & Program Design

1. **Perennial Establishment Incentives**
   - Extend existing soil & water cost-share programs to include nut-tree agroforestry (e.g., $1,000–$1,500/acre establishment grants).
   - Offer low-interest revolving loans for the 8-year maturation period.
2. **Processing & Cooperative Infrastructure**
   - Fund pilot-scale regional chestnut hubs (aggregation, drying, milling, cold storage).
   - Prioritize cooperative ownership and veteran/farmer participation.
3. **Research & Demonstration Orchards**
   - Partner with land-grant universities and state agencies to launch multi-site demonstration orchards measuring soil carbon, hydrology, and mental-health outcomes.
4. **Community Health Integration**
   - Support land-based therapy programs through state health or veterans' agencies.
   - Recognize agroforestry as a *public-health and resilience intervention*.

## Expected Returns

- **Local job creation:** nursery, harvest, processing, and educational programming.
- 15-year IRR of **13–20 %** for orchards under cooperative marketing models.
- **Carbon and ecosystem services:** potential integration into voluntary carbon markets.
- **Social capital:** strengthened communities through shared work and place-based meaning.

## Recommended Action (2026–2030)

- Establish a **North Carolina Chestnut Initiative**: a cross-agency task force linking Agriculture, Natural Resources, and Health departments.
- Launch **3 pilot demonstration sites** in distinct ecoregions (Sandhills, Piedmont, Appalachians).
- Provide seed funding for cooperative processing feasibility studies and public outreach campaigns focused on farmers.

### Contact: Nate Crew

**The DeepRichDirt Project**
www.wagramorchard.com/deeprichdirt

nate@wagramorchard.com

www.ingramcontent.com/pod-product-compliance
Lightning Source LLC
Chambersburg PA
CBHW080428030426
42335CB00020B/2644